Successful

Surrogacy

An Intended Parents' Guide to a
Rewarding Relationship With
Their Surrogate Mother

Susan MZ Fuller

Roosevelt Academy Press, Reston

ISBN: 978-0692548-81-3

www.surrogacybydesign.com

Dedication

To Doug, without whom my surrogacy experiences could never have been a success. Much love.

The Successful Surrogacy Journal

Looking for some additional tips, inspiration, and a way to record your questions and thoughts before, during, and after your surrogacy experience?

I've put together a free companion journal just for you!

Print it out to record your thoughts in writing or type directly into the PDF—it's the perfect complement to this book.

Head to www.surrogacybydesign.com/journal to download The Successful Surrogacy Journal now!

Table of Contents

Introduction

Considering having a child through gestational surrogacy can be an intimidating, sad, scary, exciting, empowering, thrilling or nerve-racking experience; and is often every one of those things! One thing is for certain though, parenthood via surrogacy is a unique experience for everyone.

And the same is true for surrogate mothers—each experience they have with a set of intended parents is different based on personalities, geography, medical history, etc. There are no universally applicable rules that cover every surrogacy arrangement.

However, as an intended parent who may be pursuing gestational surrogacy to begin, or add to, your family, you're undoubtedly filled with questions. And you should be, of course! Surrogacy, for better and for worse, is life-changing for all parties concerned.

This guide will not answer every single question you have about gestational surrogacy, nor is it meant to. There are plenty of resources out there that can educate you about the process of surrogacy—as complex as it may seem, the mechanics of the whole thing are fairly straightforward. If you have an egg (donor or maternal), sperm (donor or paternal), a host uterus and a fertility center to provide the laboratory and medical support, achieving a surrogate pregnancy is not very complicated.

The same may not be said about the emotional and interpersonal aspects of surrogacy, though. What I hope this guide will do is provide you with some topics to think about, some questions to Ask Yourself, some questions to ask your potential or current surrogate mother, and some tips to help you achieve the best experience possible with your surrogacy arrangement.

Surrogacy can be, and often is, a beautiful experience for all parties concerned. It's my hope that with the help of this guide, you and your surrogate mother will enjoy each step of the process together as you all work as a team to make your dreams come true.

You may be wondering why am I qualified to write this book. I often refer to myself, tongue-in-cheek, as a "serial surrogate" because I've been a surrogate mother seven times and given birth to nine surrogate children (two sets of twins). I have a wide variety of surrogacy experiences to draw from!

My husband and I had our first child at the age of 28. We struggled a bit to get pregnant, and because I'm a big planner and researcher, during the months we were not getting pregnant, I looked at all the various fertility treatment options. It was then that I encountered the idea of surrogacy as a genuine treatment option for some couples, not just the subject of hyped-up, comedic or overly dramatic TV movies as it has often been portrayed.

Thankfully, we ended up getting pregnant on our own after nearly two years of trying. I enjoyed an easy, comfortable pregnancy and a quick, uncomplicated delivery. It was literally minutes after my daughter's birth that I said breathlessly to my husband "Oh my God; I can't wait to do that again!" and I was dead serious about it.

Shortly after her birth I remembered my infertility research and surrogacy and decided to look into the idea of becoming a surrogate mother myself. I mentioned it to my husband, who naturally thought I was crazy, but he relented by saying that he'd consider it when we were all done having kids of our own.

Our son was born about a year and a half later and his was another simple pregnancy and quick birth. I knew by this point that I really wanted to be a surrogate mother. I contacted a few agencies and got applications so I could find out what the process entailed.

A year later our third child was born and we felt that our family was complete. I still yearned for another pregnancy, so I contacted a local agency that handled surrogacy. The owner said that I was a good candidate, but couldn't begin the process until my daughter was finished breastfeeding.

I interviewed with the agency about a year later and was accepted into the program and was matched with my first couple about a month later. I was so excited to begin!

My first surrogacy was for a local couple and I had twin girls for them. I had an easy (as twins go!), healthy pregnancy and delivered them at 39 weeks gestation. They were 6lbs and 6.9lbs at birth. I delivered the first twin vaginally with no anesthesia and I delivered the second twin by emergency C-section a couple of hours later. It was a physically traumatic delivery, but also an emotionally traumatic one, too.

The intended parents and I did not grow close during the surrogacy, and the delivery only pushed us farther apart. I've not seen the babies since I gave birth to them and they haven't stayed in touch. This hurt me deeply.

I recovered well from the difficult delivery and was ready to try again for a new couple before too long. Because I participated in a few online forums for surrogates, I knew my bad experience with the intended parents was not typical. I'd read about plenty of loving, joyous surrogacy experiences and was determined to experience that for myself.

My second surrogacy was for a local couple and I had twin boys for them. I had another easy pregnancy, though this one was a bit less comfortable because when the boys were born at 37.5 weeks, they weighted 7.8lbs and 7.9lbs. Because both babies were positioned transverse (sideways) in my belly, we had a C-section, though we waited for labor to begin rather than scheduling it ahead of time. Their birth was as wonderful and joyous as I had hoped and we've remained close ever since.

My third surrogacy was for another local couple and I carried a single girl for them. It was an easy pregnancy and an uncomplicated vaginal delivery on her due date and we're still in touch—we all enjoyed the experience together.

My fourth surrogacy was for a local couple who already had one child, but due to medical reasons, the mother was unable to carry again. After a healthy and easy pregnancy, I delivered a baby girl for them at their home. It was a lovely experience to have a planned, midwife-assisted homebirth with them. I stayed at their house for a few days, nursing the baby on demand, and pumped breast milk for her for several months.

My fifth surrogacy was for the same couple. We conceived another single girl and planned another homebirth for her. At the 20-week ultrasound, though, we found out that she had a congenital and fatal heart defect and the remainder of the pregnancy was uncertain. She passed away in utero at 24 weeks and I delivered her stillborn in the hospital. It was an emotionally painful experience as you can imagine, yet healing and reverent after being told of her diagnosis a month prior. The family has since moved from the area but we're still in touch.

My sixth surrogacy was for a gay couple, also local, and I delivered a single girl for them. Gay marriage became legal during our pregnancy so my husband and I attended their wedding—a huge celebration—when I was eight months pregnant. I delivered their baby on her due date and nursed her throughout our hospital stay. We're sporadically in touch now, and they've since had a second daughter with another surrogate.

My seventh and final surrogacy was for a couple who lives about two hours away, the farthest I've ever lived from a couple for whom I've carried. They had one child via a different surrogate, and had a harrowing experience with that surrogacy. They were a very lovely couple who truly deserved a beautiful surrogacy experience after their first one and I'm pleased to say this was indeed, an exceptional experience we enjoyed together. I delivered a healthy baby boy for them, on his due date, and we're still close.

What I've learned over the years is that there is a rich range of surrogacy experiences that one person can have, and all combined, they make for a lot of information! My goal is to pass on bits that I've learned throughout the years to help you have the best possible experience with your gestational surrogate. Your journey toward parenthood or expansion of your family will be uniquely your own, but perhaps I can help make it a little smoother and/or less stressful for all of you.

This guide is structured to take you through the surrogacy process from start to finish; beginning with the first step of deciding whether or not surrogacy is actually something you want to pursue, all the way through the birth of your baby and beyond. It hits on the key points of each phase, giving you an idea of issues you can expect to encounter and a glimpse into what your surrogate's experience may be throughout. No one can adequately capture gestational surrogacy in a way that's universally true, but based on my own experiences, I hope to offer you enough insight into the process to have the best possible relationship and results from gestational surrogacy.

And if you haven't already, I highly recommend you download the free companion journal I made to go with this book—it highlights all of the steps you'll read about here and gives you space to record your own thoughts, feelings and questions along the way so you'll be prepared for each step of the process. I've also included some bonus tips and inspiration that you won't find in this book. You can download The Successful Surrogacy Journal at www.surrogacybydesign/journal.

Deciding to Use a Gestational Surrogate

For a lot of women, realizing that they need to use a surrogate mother can be a difficult revelation to process and come to terms with, and understandably so. Some women find out early in their lives that they're unable to carry a baby, so they have many years to get used to the idea and accept it. Others find out much later, often after their own failed fertility treatments, and it becomes a last straw before pursuing adoption or choosing to remain childless.

Depending on where you are along the process of finding out you need to use a surrogate mother will determine how the following questions and tips apply to you.

Have you grieved the loss of your fertility yet?

Some women are able to move fairly quickly from the notion of being pregnant themselves to having someone else carry for them, while some women need more time to work through their range of emotions. There is no timeline that applies to all, or even most, women—it's a uniquely individual process. I encourage you to explore this issue with yourself, until you're able to feel good about using a surrogate; use others or a counselor as a sounding board if necessary. You may not resolve all of your feelings of sadness or loss, of course—that's natural—but it's key to enter into a relationship with any surrogate mother, feeling more excited about the idea of becoming a mother through alternate means, rather than feeling overwhelmed by grief over what you cannot do for yourself.

Any good surrogate understands that her intended mother will have a variety of emotions about the pregnancy and should do her best to be sensitive to her intended mother's feelings, but surrogates also want to, and generally expect to, share their pregnancy experience with her intended parents.

Ask Yourself: Am I in a mental and emotional state of mind where I can support a surrogate mother and enjoy, through her, the pregnancy as it develops?

Is your partner equally supportive of using a surrogate mother?

Pregnancy and childbirth are very intimate things to experience, and no longer will it just be you and your partner journeying through the next nine months. Your partners on this journey include not only your surrogate, but her partner if she has one, her children (which she should have, because rarely does any fertility center allow someone to be a surrogate mother without at least one previous pregnancy and delivery), and family members and friends, (both yours and the surrogate's), who will naturally be curious about the arrangement.

Both partners do not have to be equally enthusiastic or in search of an equal amount of contact or intimacy with the surrogate. However, both partners must respect and support what the other partner wants and needs from the experience. It's not about equality across the board, rather it's about respecting and supporting everyone's desires so that all needs can be met.

Ask Yourself: Are both partners open to starting or growing a family using a surrogate mother, without blame or resentment toward the intended mother who cannot carry for herself?

Have you discussed with your partner how you see yourself working with a surrogate mother?

There are lots of different possible arrangements for surrogacy, which include:

- Having a family member or close friend carry for you (usually without a fee, though you will most likely be expected to cover any surrogacy-related expenses such as out-of-pocket medical bills, child care for doctors' appointments, vitamins, maternity clothes, etc.).

- Having a local stranger carry for you (for a fee, and arranged through an agency or independently)

- Having a stranger from another part of the country carry for you (again, fee-based and arranged either through an agency or independently)

- Having an international stranger carry for you (fee-based and arranged through an agency).

Naturally there are benefits and drawbacks to each of the possibilities, and the logistics of your surrogacy arrangement will have a significant impact on how your relationship develops throughout the pregnancy (though this is not universally true, some intended parents and surrogates achieve a very close relationship even though there is great distance between them). But distance will play a role in how often you're able to see your surrogate mother, attend doctors' appointments, touch her belly and feel the baby move, etc.—so it's worthwhile exploring these issues prior to searching for a surrogate. Discuss them with your partner—while you may be okay with a surrogate five states away, your partner may feel strongly about working with someone whom you can see more often and be able to attend every doctor's appointment.

Also, consider what your long-term expectations are for your relationship with your surrogate. Do you hope to become lifelong friends, or are you seeking more of a short-term solution to your fertility problems? Either one of those, or something in between, is perfectly fine—this is your life, your baby, and your journey to parenthood. And of course, relationships can change over time, it's only natural. But, if you can articulate now what you see your ideal relationship with a surrogate mother looking like, you'll have a better chance of finding a good match with a woman who wants a similar experience for herself.

Ask Yourself: In an ideal scenario, what would my relationship with my surrogate look like? Do I want something close, with plenty of in-person contact, or would I prefer a bit more distance, with periodic updates via phone, text or email?

Do you have the financial security to use a surrogate mother?

In an ideal world, everyone would be able to get pregnant easily and every pregnancy would end with the delivery of a healthy baby (or two). But unfortunately we know that the world is less than ideal, and that's particularly true for the world of infertility treatments. It's all very expensive, plain and simple.

Even if you have great insurance coverage for IVF (lucky you!), unless your surrogate is a family member or close friend, you will have to compensate her for her time, energy and service. There is a wide range of fees that surrogates expect (you can find these numbers with some basic internet research), and you should acquaint yourself with this range.

There are a lot of different factors that determine how a surrogate sets her fee, including how experienced she is (i.e, how many previous surrogacies she's completed), the extent of her medical insurance coverage (a woman may ask for a higher fee if she has excellent maternity insurance with little-to-no out-of-pocket medical costs to her intended parents), and just plain personal preference.

Prior to looking for a surrogate mother, consider your own financial picture and make sure that you are secure enough to cover the necessary medical costs of IVF (including the egg retrieval from either the intended mother or an egg donor), health insurance for your surrogate if she doesn't have a policy that covers surrogate pregnancy, any co-pays or fees not covered by insurance, life insurance for your surrogate, and other miscellaneous expenses (usually, but not limited to, fees for cycling/embryo transfer regardless if a pregnancy is achieved, a maternity clothing allowance, additional fees for twins or triplets, a fee for undergoing a cesarean section, etc.). All of these costs are in addition to your surrogate's base fee for the pregnancy and delivery.

There is always the chance that your surrogate will be confined to bedrest because of medical complications of the pregnancy. If this is the case, you will have to pay for her lost wages if she has a job, or childcare/housekeeping expenses, or all of the above. Though no one goes into surrogacy expecting a complicated or difficult pregnancy, it can and does happen, so it's crucial that you have the financial reserves to handle any unforeseen expenses that crop up.

Ask Yourself: Are my partner and I financially secure enough to cover the cost of a surrogate pregnancy, including a reserve fund to cover unanticipated expenses? Are we both fully in favor of allocating this large sum of money toward having a baby?

Searching for a Surrogate Mother

When you decide that your best option to have a baby is using the services of a surrogate mother, it can feel overwhelming to think about how you might find someone. Could there be any job that's more important than growing and delivering your baby? Probably not!

Thankfully there are healthy and compassionate women out there who are very qualified to carry a baby for you. With careful planning and forethought, it can be a wonderful experience for all parties involved. Trust me when I say that there's nothing that thrills a surrogate mother more than seeing her intended mother hold her baby for the very first time—it's an unreal and extremely satisfying experience.

There are a number of things to keep in mind when you are seeking out a surrogate.

Do you want to use an agency to match you with a surrogate, or would you prefer to look independently?

The biggest reason why intended parents choose to work with an agency is convenience and peace of mind. The agency should do a preliminary screening of all women who apply with them to be a surrogate and only accept into their program those who show excellent potential. They should conduct a background check, a basic medical check, and a general screening of the woman's motivations for being a surrogate (money as a main motivator is frowned upon) as well as her family and living situation, to make sure she's at a stable point in her life.

Most agencies will also collect additional preference information from their potential surrogates, such as if they're open to carrying for a couple of another race, religion, or sexual orientation, under what (if any) circumstances they would consent or not consent to pregnancy termination, if they will work with only local couples, etc.

If you choose to go with an agency, they will match you only with candidates that are a fit for your requirements or wishes, as well as a surrogate whose fee is in the range you are able to pay. Experienced surrogates often have higher fees than first-time surrogates, but you also benefit from her experience and success from her previous surrogacies.

Generally speaking, an agency will also walk you through all the other legal and procedural requirements for your surrogacy arrangement. They can arrange for your psychological and medical screenings, they will prepare your legal agreement with your surrogate (or refer you to someone who will), and they will guide you along the process of the legal paperwork that accompanies your baby's birth. Some agencies even periodically monitor the surrogate's health and experience during the pregnancy in order to prevent or diffuse any potential problems. And should a serious disagreement arise between you and your surrogate during the course of the pregnancy, the agency will step in to help resolve it.

There's no question that using an agency to find your surrogate mother can be an expensive choice. However, some people feel that the peace of mind and guidance an agency can offer along the way is well worth this cost.

Some intended parents prefer to find a surrogate to carry for them on their own, and there's no question that with the help of the Internet, it can be done (and is done quite routinely). Parents who go this route may feel like they have more control over the process and can move at their own pace, rather than waiting for an agency to have the time or resources to match them. Most often intended parents will place ads on surrogacy websites and potential surrogates will get in touch to begin the screening process.

Usually this contact and screening is done via email, and then evolves to telephone calls, and finally face-to-face meetings.

Should you find a suitable match this way, you will then be responsible for arranging your own medical and psychological screenings and working with an attorney to prepare the legal agreement and establish an escrow account to disburse regular payments to your surrogate.

From the surrogate's perspective, there are various reasons why she may use an agency versus attempting an independent agreement. She may opt for an agency for the same reasons you might—she has one point of contact for all of the various steps in the process, she does not have to do the legwork of communicating with various couples in search of a match, she does not have to negotiate agreement details directly with the intended parents, and the couples the agency offers to match her with are also pre-screened.

Women who choose to pursue surrogacy independently may do so because they've had experience as a surrogate and feel they can handle all the components on their own, or because they wish to offer potential couples a more cost-effective alternative, or because perhaps there are no agencies near them (though most agencies work with surrogates from all over the country). Be aware though, that a surrogate who is pursuing an independent agreement could be someone who was not accepted to work with an agency for any number of reasons (health, psychological, socio-economic, etc.). This, to be certain, applies to the minority of women choosing to go the independent route, but it's worth mentioning and considering if you pursue an independent surrogacy arrangement.

Ask Yourself: Does the idea of working with an agency give me peace of mind because I know there is another party walking us through the process and vouching for the quality of the potential surrogates I'll be matched with, or am I an independent person who would rather take things at my own speed and manage all the various components myself?

Other than good health, mental stability and a successful pregnancy and delivery history, what are some important qualities you're looking for in a surrogate mother?

Everyone, intended parents and surrogates alike, has an ideal match in mind. And "ideal" is exactly that—a wish list of characteristics, skills, or experiences that you'd love to find in one person, in a perfect world.

But, we all know we don't live in a perfect world (if we did, there'd be no need for surrogate mothers), so the best approach you can take is to create a list of factors you think are most important, and another list of factors that would be nice to have, but you don't think are absolutely critical.

If you are using an agency to find a surrogate, be sure to be upfront with them about your list of "must haves"— they can't read your mind! Maybe your requirements relate to geography—how far away your surrogate lives— or maybe you definitely want a surrogate who is married. If there's something on your mind that feels just right to you, acknowledge it by putting it on the list.

If you're searching for a surrogate on your own, you'll need to be more thorough in your screening because no one is doing the initial vetting for you. You'll want to develop a list of basic screening questions to weed out women who are obviously not a good fit for you before moving onto more specific, personal attributes you're looking for.

If you have any non-negotiable things on your list (for example, you will only transfer one embryo at a time because you want to reduce your chances of multiples), be sure to tell any potential surrogate mothers about it early on in the screening process to avoid wasting both of your time, in case she does not feel the same way as you do on the topic.

Even if you're largely flexible with what you're looking for in a surrogate mother, it's a useful exercise to get down on paper the qualities your ideal surrogate would possess and what your ideal surrogacy experience would look like. Knowing the things that are most important to you can help guide future conversations with potential surrogates.

Ask Yourself: How would I describe to a friend the ideal surrogate mother to carry my baby? What qualities would she possess?

What type of surrogacy experience are you looking to have?

While you may think that it's too hard to determine this without any prior surrogacy experience, it's worth the time and effort to think things over and formulate some thoughts about your expectations before you start. Are you looking for a close, almost sister-like relationship with your surrogate mother? Or do you envision something that's closer to a business arrangement where your contact is limited to periodic reports throughout the pregnancy, and you don't expect to maintain much, if any, contact after the birth? Or maybe you hope it's something in between the two?

If you are hoping to limit your contact throughout the pregnancy, and especially after the birth of your child or children, it's only fair that you express this early on in the getting-to-know-you phase of things. There is nothing wrong if this is how you'd like your surrogacy to be—this is your experience and you deserve to feel good about it. But be forewarned that most surrogates aren't doing this for the money—they're primarily motivated by the idea of helping another woman reach her dream of becoming a mother or a male couple become fathers. And at least for every surrogate mother I know, there's little that's more rewarding than getting pictures and updates on the baby she brought into the world.

As with any other relationship, feelings grow and change over time and this is completely natural. Personally speaking, I keep in closer touch with some intended parents more than others and I have the least contact with some that I'm closest with—we all have busy families that leave us with little time to catch up. But when we do, we're instantly close again. That's something that I wanted from each of my surrogacies and something I made sure my intended parents wanted as well.

After my first rocky surrogacy experience, I learned to ask about this explicitly when interviewing with potential intended parents. The women you talk with may or may not think to ask about the future—but it's worth it to all of you to think through and talk about how you'd like the relationship to develop over time (or not, as the case may be). When it comes to surrogacy, there might be one golden rule—the fewer surprises, the better!

Ask Yourself: How do I see my surrogate mother fitting into my life both during the pregnancy and afterward?

Can you trust your gut?

Surrogacy is a very emotional and personal process that can be only regulated by procedures and tests and contracts so much. Doctors and science can guide you on many, but not all, things, and you will have to trust your gut reaction and intuition when choosing a surrogate mother to carry your baby.

Take into account how you feel getting to know her, whether she seems organized and forthcoming, or whether you have to pull information out of her. Is she prompt with her reply emails or texts? Here's a caveat though—be sure to take into account that all surrogates are mothers themselves, and many of them have young children who require a lot of their time and attention. Therefore, they may not be as quick to reply to requests as you might be—this is just a reality of the demands of motherhood. However, anyone who is looking to be a surrogate mother should be timely the majority of the time and if not, you should give hard consideration to whether or not she's a good fit for you.

I'd invite you to consider how much you trust your intuition, and how much your partner trusts his or hers. Does one of you seem to have instincts that are more spot-on than the other? Then make sure that person is actively involved in deciding whether or not to work with a particular person as your surrogate mother.

You might describe this as that infamous "click" you feel with someone—that's a good thing! That's a definite bonus if you feel that "click." But definitely make sure everything else checks out medically, psychologically, etc. before entering into a surrogacy agreement and making plans for an embryo transfer.

And what if everything does check out, and everything seems good on paper, but you have that little voice inside you raising doubts? My best advice to you is to listen to it. If you're one who often says to yourself "I should have listened to myself when I thought…." then now is not the time to ignore your inner voice.

A lot of the process of surrogacy is about science and law and facts and procedures, but an awful lot of it is also about how a surrogate mother and her intended parents function as a team. There's only so much of this you can figure out ahead of time, so you really have to learn to trust what your gut is telling you.

Ask Yourself: After many discussions and getting to know my potential surrogate mother, do I feel good about embarking on this journey with her? Do I have any unresolved, and possibly unvoiced, concerns?

Cycling and Getting Pregnant

The old saying of "hurry up and wait" might be surrogacy's biggest catch phrase. Nothing about surrogacy is quick, or at least it feels that way. Everyone is so excited to keep moving forward toward their goal of having a baby, but the process can seem excruciatingly slow. And truthfully, sometimes it just is very slow because of all the physical, medical, and legal procedures that have to take place, often in a particular order, coordinating across numerous different professionals. It can be a real juggling act and most of the time, unfortunately, there just aren't a lot of ways to speed things up.

As you get to this point with your surrogate, undoubtedly all of you will be getting more and more excited to get the show on the road, so to speak. So much preparation goes into getting here and now you're finally onto the business of getting pregnant!

This phase also gives you another chance to bond with your surrogate mother as an individual person (rather than just as the woman who's carrying your baby) and vice versa—she will have time to get to know you better—which will definitely help things go more smoothly when you're sharing a pregnancy together.

How has your communication been until this point? Are you satisfied with it, or do you feel you want more or less communication with your surrogate?

Of course everyone wants their relationships to develop and evolve naturally, but in many ways surrogacy doesn't quite fit the definition of natural—two people can go from absolute strangers to connected in the most intimate way in just a matter of months. While in most situations this is a positive development, it's also worth some thought and introspection along the way.

Whether this is your surrogate's first experience or her fifth, each step along the way is as exciting to her as it is for you, no doubt. Not only is she adding components to her daily routine (whether taking pills or using patches or suppositories or doing shots, or all of the above) which require some lifestyle adjustment, she's now taking some form of hormones. That's significant for a woman who is probably in the throes of mothering her own children, too (or even if she's not).

Your surrogate would probably think it's thoughtful of you to check in at each phase of the cycling protocol, asking her how the shots are going or if she's feeling any side effects from the oral medication, etc. Most surrogates are eager to share their experience with their intended mother (or both intended parents too, if you tend to communicate as a couple to her) and so if you ask, she'll most likely think it to be more thoughtful rather than an intrusion.

If there are certain days or times or benchmarks when you'd like your surrogate mother to check in with you, by all means, tell her. She wants to make this a good experience for you and by letting her know what you'd like from her in the way of communication, it will only help your relationship grow.

But also consider that she is probably a busy mother herself, as most surrogates are still caring for their own children as they carry babies for their intended parents. And aside from keeping up with her medical protocol or a sudden medical emergency, caring for her family should always come first—there may very well be times that she doesn't have the time or energy to devote to a long conversation, and it's important to respect that. In this case, you could ask her for a brief check-in and then schedule a time later for a longer catch-up.

Ask Yourself: Am I satisfied with the frequency and quality of communication with my surrogate mother, and if not, how can I change that? If I look as objectively as possible from my surrogate's point of view, is there a better way I can support her, either through more or possibly less contact with her?

Do you feel you know your surrogate as a person apart from her role as your surrogate mother? What can you do now to further that understanding?

It might seem obvious to say, but your surrogate is more than the host uterus for your baby and more than the mother to her own children. Of course she must love pregnancy and mothering to want to be a surrogate in the first place, and that's the bond that will tie you together. But she's also a woman with a family of origin, a spouse (most likely in some form, even if she's not married), a career or work history prior to her becoming a mother, hobbies and just general interests (music, reading, sports, home decorating, etc.)

She probably wanted to know all about you when deciding to carry for you because it's important for her to feel confident and happy about where the baby she carries will end up. And undoubtedly you asked her about herself and her interests as well. But there's a chance that in all the excitement of meeting and deciding whether or not you were "a match," you didn't absorb a lot about her as her own person—the things she enjoys aside from her life as a mother and as the role of a potential surrogate. And of course that's natural—those early days and weeks are so exciting and full of questions and information, there's no way you can explore everything about each other.

So while you're going through your pre-transfer cycle or even during your 2-week wait (the name used for the time between the embryo transfer and the blood pregnancy test), it's nice to have other ways to engage with one another besides focusing exclusively on the anticipated pregnancy. That might be through common interests, or just getting more familiar with each other's interests and hobbies by asking and chatting about things important or enjoyable to your surrogate, but unrelated to surrogacy.

This will not only help pass the time during your pre-transfer cycling and 2-week wait (both of which seem to take much, much longer than the calendar says it should), it will also give you a richer, more solid foundation for your relationship during the pregnancy and afterward. Although it's everyone's goal to grow a family, everyone also likes to be understood and appreciated as individuals, as well.

Ask Yourself: Have I taken the time to genuinely get to know my surrogate, apart from her role in growing my family? Do I find ways to engage with and acknowledge her as an individual so she feels valued as a person, not just for her role as a surrogate mother?

What can you do to show your surrogate mother your appreciation for undergoing the transfer and the rest time afterward?

As mentioned previously, as you're cycling and preparing for the embryo transfer, your surrogate will probably appreciate casual check-ins from you asking how she's doing with each new medication or step in the process. No need to hover or be overbearing or even overly appreciative of course, but knowing that you're thinking of her and recognizing the steps she's taking along the way will help her feel that you're all in this together and this is a team effort.

By the time the transfer arrives, you're all getting very excited, and understandably so! While the transfer itself is rather quick and painless (except for the overly full bladder your surrogate will have—that part is no fun), the next few hours, days, and weeks will be fraught with wonder and anticipation and even worry for all of you. This is all completely normal, of course.

The days of extended post-transfer bedrest have long passed. However, most fertility centers request (or even require) a surrogate to take it easy for a day or two after the transfer. This will probably mean your surrogate will camp out on the couch for a while, or if she has small children who might not understand why mommy isn't down on the floor giving horsey rides like usual, she may be holed up in her bedroom for the majority of the time. Some intended parents even put the surrogate up in a hotel, not only to ensure she's getting peaceful rest, but to indulge her in a little pampering.

Regardless of how your surrogate spends her post-transfer rest time, it's nice to offer her a gesture of your appreciation. Paying for her hotel stay and meals is one way, of course, but it need not be that grand if that's not something that works for you (and it may not work for her). Sending her home from the transfer with some prepared meals she can provide her family is very thoughtful and greatly appreciated, not to mention very practical since her family needs to eat whether she's been ordered to rest on the couch or not. Or giving her a gift card or certificates for local carry-out food works, or even something as simple as sending a fruit basket for everyone to nibble on.

Of course your main goal is to take care of and show appreciation for your surrogate, but there's no denying that surrogacy is a family affair affecting everyone your surrogate is close to, particularly her husband and children. They may be just as excited as you are for her to get pregnant, but there's no question that there are times over the long haul that the glow of the surrogacy experience wears thin. Letting everyone in her family know that you recognize and appreciate what they're all going through does a lot to keep everyone focused on the end goal—a happy and healthy pregnancy that results in a healthy baby.

Other things you may consider for your surrogate during this time are books, magazines, DVDs or online subscriptions to help her pass the time, bath and body products for her to pamper herself with, a piece of jewelry to remind her that you're thinking of her (it needn't be expensive, just something that you think she'll enjoy or something that's symbolic to her), etc.

If possible, let her take the lead on communicating with you during this time. While she's under orders to rest (and particularly if she had to take tranquilizers for the transfer, as is protocol for some fertility centers), she just might be catching up on her sleep and you don't want to be the one to wake her up! A simple text or email letting her know that you're thinking of her and wishing her the best is always appreciated and helps bridge the gap until your next, more in-depth, conversation.

Ask Yourself: Am I doing my best to balance my own need to connect with my surrogate mother with her possible need for quiet and space during this exciting and stressful time? How can I help her support her family when she's not able to attend to all their needs?

Do you have strong feelings about your surrogate mother taking home pregnancy tests?

Ah, the hot topic of home pregnancy tests. Either you love them or you hate them, there's little ground in between. Chances are, though, that your surrogate loves them. And that's okay, even if you hate them. There's definitely a middle ground you can find.

Fertility centers often caution against them because the results are not as definitive as the beta hCG blood test they do. While this is true, most beta hCG blood tests aren't done until at least 10 days after the embryo transfer, and sometimes more. It can be a long, agonizing wait for everyone to find out if the transfer worked.

Assuming that you're using a gestational surrogate, a positive home pregnancy test will show that some changes are happening (or not) with the embryo, though it won't provide you any qualitative measure of how successful the pregnancy might be.

Talk with your surrogate about whether or not she wants to do home tests. Most surrogates want to do them, so no need to feel like you have to tread lightly with this topic. She's probably expecting you to ask about it. And definitely be honest about your feelings on the topic.

If you want her to do home testing, then feel free to stock her up with a wide variety of tests—she will greatly appreciate that. The tests are pricey and many surrogates find doing a range of tests over several days or a week to be a real treat.

If you don't want her to do home testing, let her know that, too, and she just might agree with you (though this would be the exception to the rule). If you truly don't want to know until you get the results of her beta hCG blood test, it's better to tell her not to tell you the results, should she decide to take a home test (or two or three or more).

While it's reasonable for you to want to wait for the definitive blood test results, it's not entirely reasonable to ask her to wait as well. She's the one who's still keeping up with her medication protocol and feeling the side effects, while totally uncertain if they're caused by all the drugs, or it's the beginning of a pregnancy. She may find taking home pregnancy tests exciting and reassuring.

If you are certain that you don't want to know any results until the blood test, then be clear about that with her. Let her know that if she chooses to test at home, under no circumstances should she let you know the results, positive or negative. No need to be harsh or critical about it (in fact, quite the contrary), just respect that you two might feel differently on the issue of testing and politely ask her to respect your wishes.

Ask Yourself: How do I want to find out the results of our embryo transfer? Would I prefer to hear earlier, based on the results of home pregnancy tests (recognizing that they're not 100% certain) or would I rather wait to get the definitive numerical results from the beta hCG blood tests?

The Pregnancy

Congratulations, you're pregnant! You've gotten past all the preparations and cycling and transfer and two-week wait and you've found out that you're expecting a baby (or maybe two). The nine months ahead of you will probably fly by with all the excitement.

Early in the pregnancy is a good time to reflect on how you feel the surrogacy experience has been going so far. Hopefully you and your surrogate are building a positive relationship with each other that will continue to strengthen throughout the pregnancy. But also given the length of time of the pregnancy and the long stretches of not much to report (particularly early on when doctor's appointments are a month or more apart) you may not be in as close touch as you were prior to getting pregnant. That's all part of the natural ebb and flow, of course, and things will pick up again as the pregnancy progresses. Your relationship will grow and change in many ways, as it will once your baby is in your arms. Knowing what to expect can make the experience richer for all of you.

How much do you want to know about the pregnancy symptoms your surrogate is experiencing?

Because they aren't able to carry the baby for themselves, some intended mothers want to hear absolutely everything about the pregnancy experience, and that's understandable. Sharing the progression of the pregnancy through your surrogate's descriptions and updates can be a vital link to bonding with your baby before he or she is born.

Most surrogates (like most people in general) are happy to talk about how they're feeling, so don't hesitate to ask. It's expected that a surrogate will check in with you after each doctor's appointment, if you're not able to attend them with her. This is a natural opportunity for you to learn about what she's currently going through and to catch up with each other.

As a general rule, surrogates will offer a lot of information and most will welcome endless questions, though some women are just more private by nature. If your surrogate isn't as forthcoming with information as you hoped, be aware that sometimes a surrogate hesitates to offer information to her intended mother because she doesn't want her to feel bad. She's keenly aware of the loss component of surrogacy and she may be treading lightly to avoid exacerbating possible feelings of grief in her intended mother.

Ask your surrogate mother about how she's feeling in general, as well as questions specific to the pregnancy or things you're curious about. One thing to be mindful of though is how your questions might be perceived—be sure that they're coming from a place of genuine concern and curiosity rather than as a means of "checking up" on your surrogate to make sure she's doing things to your standards (unless you have a reason to believe she's being reckless, in which case it's an issue to address with your agency, the doctor, or her directly). Keep in mind that just like you, it's your surrogate's goal to have a healthy, comfortable pregnancy and delivery—you are all in this for the same reason.

Your own feelings of loss during the pregnancy are completely normal, even though you are thrilled that your surrogate is pregnant and you're closer to being parents, either for the first time, or again. It's understandable and natural to feel both excited and disappointed about the pregnancy, but hopefully you're able to still enjoy sharing the experience through your surrogate's updates.

If it's truly difficult for you to talk about the pregnancy with her, it's worth seeking out counseling to better understand your own feelings and find constructive ways to work through them. This is in your own best interest, as well as the best interest of your surrogate mother, and ultimately your baby. Getting to a place where everyone is as comfortable and open as possible is a goal everyone should agree on so don't be afraid to pursue it.

Ask Yourself: How can I find a balance between what I want to know about the pregnancy and what our surrogate wants to share? Do both I and my surrogate mother seem comfortable with the flow of information between you about the pregnancy?

How aligned is your personality with your surrogate's?

There is nothing that will bond you to your surrogate mother like sharing the experience of having a baby together. Just by its very nature, your relationship has the potential to be very close.

Hopefully, during the process of deciding to work together you were able to gauge how similar and how different your personalities are from each other, so there aren't any big surprises now that you're expecting a baby. But life does happen and circumstances do change, so your relationship may not be exactly what you expected it to be. And don't underestimate the power of hormones, either—yours or your surrogate's. Your surrogate is experiencing a flood of pregnancy hormones that are constantly fluctuating beyond her control, so you may need to be extra sensitive to that.

Just take things day-by-day and week-by-week, allowing things to grow naturally. You need not be best friends throughout the pregnancy or afterward (though you very well might end up that way). Acknowledging that you're both undertaking something special and learning and growing together through this nine months is often enough to draw you close over time.

And if you don't end up growing very close, that's OK, too. The main goal of gestational surrogacy is to bring a very much loved and wanted child into the world—not to make a new best friend. Respect the natural development of your relationship and respect each other above all, and let the rest naturally evolve.

Ask Yourself: When matching with my surrogate mother, was I honest about our personalities and how our relationship might grow over time? If a gap exists in our current relationship, what can I do to bridge it, while being true to myself and sensitive to my surrogate's personality?

How are you recognizing your surrogate as a person and how her roles as a wife and mother are affected by surrogacy?

It's true that the whole reason that your surrogate mother is in your life is for the purpose of carrying your baby—for most intended parents and surrogates, that's what's drawn you together. However, even before becoming your surrogate, she was a mother and (most likely) a wife.

She maintains these roles throughout the pregnancy as well, and there's no question that the pregnancy affects her entire family. In many ways this is a positive effect of course (and if you're seeking a surrogate without the help of an agency, that's one thing you should look into in depth—how her husband and children feel about the prospect of sharing her with a couple who are virtual strangers). With any luck, her husband and children will enjoy being part of this miraculous experience.

Keep in mind, though, that along with carrying your child, your surrogate is also taking care of her own children and attending to the special events that are significant to her family life—holidays, birthdays, special celebrations. Whether planned and predetermined or not, she needs to consider and allow for how the pregnancy will affect her family obligations.

Most women think these things through prior to entering into a surrogacy agreement or consenting to a transfer schedule, but sometimes the unforeseen comes up. She may not have known nine months ahead of time that her siblings were planning a 50th anniversary party for their parents on the opposite coast, just weeks from her due date, which now she can not attend. Life just happens that way sometimes.

Taking care to recognize special dates and events that happen during the pregnancy will go a long way toward making your surrogate feel appreciated. Although her husband's birthday or her child's graduation aren't special to you, recognizing that she's participating in them while pregnant with your child is thoughtful. There's no need to go overboard, a simple card or text or email is usually enough (use your judgment—if her child is graduating from high school during the pregnancy, it's thoughtful to send a little something in recognition, but for the average birthday or celebration, your well wishes are probably enough).

Once your surrogate's pregnant belly is obvious to others, your child in utero is part of her daily life and any special event she attends, whether she wants it to be the case or not—there's just no way around it for her (and sometimes she might not want it to be—the surrogacy aspect can be an unwelcome distraction in some settings). Appreciating that she's taking part in her family life with your new family member along for the ride is a considerate thing to do.

Ask Yourself: How can I acknowledge and support my surrogate mother's personal and family life, now that the pregnancy with my baby is an added factor to her everyday reality?

How much involvement would she like from you in tasks that are hers to complete? (e.g. selecting doctors, requesting tests, completing paperwork, etc.)

Ultimately, it's your surrogate mother's responsibility to manage all the administrative tasks related to the pregnancy, and many things are much easier for her to do herself, such as making appointments that fit her schedule. You should expect her to attend to the administrative details in a timely way. She may be very happy to take care of everything herself and just update you along the way.

You could, however, offer to help her with any tasks you think you're able to, such as tracking down a notary for legal forms, or finding a lab that does the test she needs, or scheduling bloodwork, etc. Or you can ask her if she'd like reminders for tasks that are on a deadline. While she may not need or want these, she will probably find the gesture to be thoughtful and it's another way for you to feel more involved in the pregnancy.

Ask Yourself: Am I willing and able to assist with some of the administrative tasks and paperwork that come along with pregnancy, if my surrogate mother would like help?

Are there ways you can help if your surrogate runs into administrative trouble (scheduling tests, getting referrals, getting reimbursements, etc)?

While surrogacy is becoming more commonplace and the processes and procedures are much more clearly defined than in years past, there may still be times where things don't go according to plan when your surrogate tries to set things up or make arrangements. In some cases she'll be obligated to take care of things herself (such as getting medical records) and there's nothing you can do, but there may be times you can lend a hand.

Offering to help her work through red tape (and there always seems to be something that pops up) lets her know that you care about not only your baby, but her as a person and her experience along the way. Sometimes just listening to her vent her frustration or voice her concerns is enough, so offer her your ear if there's nothing you can do to help resolve it. It will help your relationship grow and may even help her think of new ways to approach and resolve the issue.

Ask Yourself: When unexpected snags come up, in what ways can I help, even if it's just listening and offering suggestions?

How can you share, with her, your own preparations for the baby—classes you're taking, pictures of the nursery, shopping, etc.?

Just as you probably enjoy seeing your surrogate mother's belly grow and feeling the baby kick when you visit, she will most likely enjoy hearing and seeing how you're preparing for life with your new baby. Just because she's not interested in adding to her own family doesn't mean she won't find it enjoyable and satisfying to share in the excitement as she is growing your new little one.

If you're geographically close to your surrogate, it's much easier of course—she can easily visit your house and see the baby's nursery and other preparations you're making. But if you're not within easy driving distance, be sure to share pictures and other plans with her.

Don't feel like you need to solicit her opinion on decisions you're making about your baby once it comes home (unless you really want to, remember, she's probably had recent experience with the exact same things for herself, so she might be able to provide valuable input) but rather share your thoughts and plans with her. Although she's entering into the surrogacy arrangement knowing full well where her boundaries are with your baby, she will also appreciate having an accurate vision in her mind of where the baby will be after it goes home with you. And because the vast majority of surrogate mothers bond with their intended parents, not the baby itself, she will genuinely enjoy hearing about and seeing your excitement with the preparations for your baby.

Ask Yourself: Have I made time to update my surrogate mother on how we're preparing for our baby's arrival?

Have you considered including your surrogate in baby-related celebrations like showers or receptions?

There are mixed feelings on this and both are legitimate, of course. Some intended parents really embrace the teamwork aspect of surrogacy and want to include their surrogate mothers in any parties being held in honor of the baby or pregnancy. If this is the case, then definitely invite her—your surrogate will probably be touched and it's highly unlikely she'll feel burdened by the invitation.

She may opt not to come of course, either due to family obligations or not wanting to feel like the center of attention or just plain old pregnancy-related fatigue. Or, she may defer because she wants the spotlight to be on you rather than on her for a change.

Also related to the pregnancy spotlight, some intended mothers would rather celebrate without their surrogate mothers present for privacy reasons, or if they still have unresolved feelings of loss over not being able to carry themselves. Of course this is fine, everyone has to be comfortable with the arrangements and your surrogate mother would never want you to feel uncomfortable with her presence. But if these feelings ring true for you, it might be worth exploring what you can work through to better come to peace with the arrangement—everyone usually has a better surrogacy experience when they feel like they're all working together toward a common goal.

Ask Yourself: How can I share the experience of baby-related celebrations with my surrogate mother in a way that makes us both feel comfortable and valued?

In what ways can you offer your surrogate mother small gestures of support, including for her family, throughout the pregnancy?

As time goes on through the pregnancy, it's natural that your attention will shift from your surrogate mother carrying your baby to her imminent labor and delivery and your new life as a family. And of course this is what the whole process is all about. You should be getting excited, and no doubt your surrogate mother is getting excited for you!

Even in the easiest and most non-eventful pregnancies, a pregnant woman needs extra rest and accommodation, particularly in the third trimester. That's just a natural part of any pregnancy. She may be too tired or feel too big to do a lot of cooking or cleaning, or she may not be able to do as much with her children as she'd like.

And although she may have a wonderful support system of family and friends who are happy to offer her help now and then, it's nice to acknowledge what she's going through in the late stages of pregnancy—it is exhausting, both mentally and physically, and even emotionally. Your gestures could be simple, such as lending a sympathetic ear or texting her periodically to see how she's doing, to sending her funny cards or emails, to something more elaborate like treating her to a prenatal massage or a dinner out for her family.

If this is the first surrogacy experience for your surrogate and her family, they may be feeling overwhelmed by and uncertain about the whole experience, just because the unknown can be stressful. Showing them that you're concerned about their experience as well as your own can help ease any anxious feelings on their part, thus giving your surrogate mother more peace of mind, which of course is most beneficial for your baby.

Ask Yourself: How am I able to demonstrate support and concern for my surrogate and her family as the pregnancy progresses and she is able to do less?

How can you support your surrogate mother as the delivery date draws closer and she needs to make plans for taking care of her own family while she's in the hospital?

Because it's likely that your surrogate mother has young children at home, she's probably already thought through the logistics of who will care for them when she's at the hospital, particularly when her husband or partner is with her during labor and delivery (which is not an absolute certainty, but it's the most likely scenario). And making these arrangements is her responsibility of course, not yours.

Talking through these plans with her well before her due date is a good idea, for a few reasons. First, it's a demonstration to her that you care about her whole experience with the surrogacy, which definitely includes her children's experience, not just her pregnancy.

Second, it's good to know her plans so should anything unexpected come up during the labor and hospital stay and she's unable to address it herself, you're in a position to offer information or support if needed. And third, you can be a valuable and objective set of eyes and ears for the arrangements, offering suggestions and feedback if necessary.

Finally, you'll want to know if she has plans to have her children come see her and the baby during her hospital stay. While you'll all need to remain flexible with expectations until after the birth, it's good to know up front what her plans are, so you're not surprised while wrapped up in those first few days with your newborn at the hospital.

Ask Yourself: Have I talked through with my surrogate mother how she will manage her own family responsibilities during labor and delivery?

How do you feel about how your communication with your surrogate mother has been so far throughout the pregnancy? Do you feel that you need more information and connection with her, or are you satisfied?

If at any point you feel like you're not getting as much communication as you'd like from your surrogate mother, don't be afraid to bring it up. The vast majority of surrogate mothers yearn for a close, communicative relationship with their intended parents and the fact is, relationships like that are built, not made instantly. And even if you both felt that initial spark of connection when meeting and deciding to work together, the whole surrogacy process is a long road with a lot of outside influences from everyday life going on at the same time.

Whether or not this is the first surrogacy for either of you, this is most likely the first time you two are part of this very unique relationship with each other. Both of you are probably in it not only for you to have a baby, but to really enjoy sharing a very special experience.

Some surrogate mothers can be tentative with sharing information because they want to be sensitive to their intended parents' feelings, so if you're someone who wants to know as much as possible about your surrogate's pregnancy experience, then be sure to ask her plenty of questions. Don't feel that you're asking too many questions (within reason of course—asking about her pregnancy symptoms and experiences is fine, prying into other issues in her life that aren't related to, or affecting, the pregnancy is not).

It's a very reasonable request to expect her to check in with you after each doctor's appointment (assuming you're not able to attend them yourself). She should be doing this without you asking, but in case she's not, it's fine to ask her to update you on the same day that she has appointments.

You may also consider setting regular dates and times for catch-up phone calls, especially as the pregnancy moves along and you're wrapped up in preparing for your baby and she's juggling the demands of the pregnancy, caring for her own family, and other work or family obligations. You might be surprised at how quickly time slips by for both of you, and setting a regular time to chat can be helpful to all of you.

As the pregnancy goes on it's likely you'll develop your own routines for keeping in touch, and thankfully technology makes it easier than ever before. Just remember that while technology is great, sometimes a little thoughtful planning and honest dialogue is more helpful than anything else.

Ask Yourself: Do I feel good about the amount and kind of communication I have with my surrogate mother? If not, how can I address it early on so we both have the best possible experience together?

Labor, Delivery, and the Hospital Stay

A lot of what happens during the labor, delivery and hospital stay will be dictated by the hospital policies, so it makes sense to discuss your surrogacy situation with the hospital you plan to use for the birth. Thankfully, as surrogacy becomes more common, many hospitals have become more accommodating with their policies or are open to deviating from their established protocols.

But there are always unplanned elements in even the most controlled and scheduled deliveries, so it's helpful to keep an open mind and be flexible. There are plenty of things to think through, discuss, and decide on, but understanding that sometimes birth is wildly unpredictable will help all of you stay in a positive and cooperative frame of mind despite the nerves and emotions everyone will be feeling.

Who will be present during labor? Who will be your surrogate mother's labor support person?

Most surrogates expect their husband or partner to play an active role in their labor and delivery, and understandably so. Her husband is probably the person she's closest to, has gone through at least one other labor and delivery with, and who she trusts the most. Also, her husband can probably make medical decisions on her behalf in the unlikely, but possible, event that she's not able to do so.

Some women, however, prefer to have a professional labor support person called a doula help them during their labor, or even a trusted friend or relative. If this is the case, talk to your surrogate about her expectations and how she envisions all of you working together. Labor and delivery rooms are not very spacious so it's helpful to have clear expectations for everyone's roles and responsibilities on the big day.

You should also discuss each other's expectations for your own roles during the labor and delivery. Do you hope to be part of your surrogate's support team in an active way, or will that be difficult for you, so instead you see yourself as more of a quiet observer? Either way is fine of course—there is no absolute right way, and things can change unexpectedly along the way—such is the unpredictable nature of childbirth. But to the greatest extent possible, it's helpful to share your ideas and hopes with each other beforehand, so everyone goes into the experience understanding what the others are hoping to achieve.

Flexibility is key here, too! Any number of issues can crop up with the baby, your surrogate mother, the hospital, your doctor, the equipment, etc. And truthfully, something unexpected usually does pop up that will necessitate a change in plans. With plenty of pre-birth talking and planning, you'll all be better able to take the unexpected in stride and still enjoy a successful and gratifying birth experience.

Ask Yourself: How do I hope to take part in my surrogate mother's labor—as a participant or as an observer?

Does your surrogate mother have any specific requests or rituals for her labor?

Some women have certain things that are important or comforting to them during labor and delivery, and these things can vary wildly. Some women don't want to be touched during a contraction while others find massage a helpful coping technique. Some women prefer to wear socks throughout labor and delivery while others need to be barefoot. Some find walking or talking to be a welcome distraction while others need to be still and quiet to cope with the pain. Others prefer soft music, or darkness, or wide-open shades.

To the greatest extent that you can, honor these requests during labor and delivery, because they will make your surrogate feel that much more comfortable, which will ultimately be better for you and your baby. Most surrogates want the delivery to be a pleasant experience for their intended parents, and so the more comfortable she is, the more comfortable you will be.

And by the same token, if there are particular things that are important to you during labor and delivery (music, lighting, noise, etc.) be sure to bring them up to your surrogate mother as well. Assuming that your relationship is strong, she will probably want to do her best to accommodate your wishes as well, so don't be afraid to ask.

Ask Yourself: How can you support your surrogate's labor experience in a way that feels true to yourself, and also meets your own needs for taking part in your baby's birth?

Who will be present during the baby's delivery?

The hospital may have a policy on how many people are able to be in the room during a vaginal birth (and they most definitely have one concerning cesarean births) so if you'd like to have more than just you and your partner, your surrogate's partner, and possibly a doula, you should check with the hospital you plan to use. For many people, birth is an intimate experience and they want to keep the crowd to a minimum (at least for the actual delivery) but in case you're looking for more participation, check with the hospital, and then check with your surrogate mother to find out what her thoughts and feelings are on it.

Be sure to keep an open and accommodating mind throughout the labor and delivery process—women in labor can have strong feelings and opinions and sometimes they even surprise themselves with them! No two labors or deliveries are the same, so although your surrogate might anticipate being open to a particular plan or arrangement, understand that she may feel differently at the actual time of the delivery and try to respect her wishes if you can.

If you're planning a cesarean birth, your doctor and hospital will advise you on the policy of who may be present. If it's a planned C-section, both intended parents may be able to attend the delivery along with your surrogate's husband, depending on hospital policy, your doctor's preference, and the medical circumstances.

In the case of an emergency C-section, you will have little time to think or plan—so it's best to discuss this scenario ahead of time. In the majority of cases, a surrogate will want her husband to accompany her, but not always. Some surrogates want the baby's mother to be there for the actual birth, and you should not grapple with this decision in the heat (and stress) of the moment, so talk it out well in advance of your due date so you have a plan that you all agree on.

There are some intended parents (intended fathers, mostly) who do not wish to be in the room during labor or delivery. If this is the case, it's important to discuss this with your surrogate ahead of time, so she's not taken by surprise. She could interpret this lack of involvement in her labor and delivery as lack of caring for her or the child she's about to give birth to, when that may not be the case at all, there could be many different reasons for one or both of the parents to not attend the actual delivery. It's important for all of you to have an honest conversation with each other so everyone has the same expectations prior to your surrogate going into labor.

Ask Yourself: Have you come up with a plan for who will be present for the actual delivery of the baby, in various circumstances?

For those attending the birth, where will they be?

Generally speaking, there are three different spots someone might stand during a birth, all of which offer a different experience. Although things can (and often do) change during the anticipation, chaos and joy of birth, it's worth thinking through where everyone in the room will stand.

You might want to stand near your surrogate's head so you can hold her hand, easily talk to her, or even just view the birth itself from her vantage point. When standing at your surrogate's head, you will not have a clear view of her vagina or of the baby emerging. Many intended fathers choose to stand in this position.

Another option is to stand next to her legs, so you have a clear view of your baby being born. Many surrogates are completely comfortable with both their intended mother and father standing here to view the birth, while others prefer that the intended father (or even both intended parents) stay near her head to offer her more privacy. It's important to ask about and respect your surrogate mother's wishes for modesty.

If you are standing near her legs, the nurse or doctor may ask you to hold one of her legs to help her push the baby out, and this is a way that many intended parents are able to participate in their baby's birth. Again, your surrogate may feel too modest for you to do this, or she may welcome your participation—it's an important topic to broach well in advance of the birth.

The remaining option for viewing the birth is from a bit of a distance, such as the other side of the room. This might be preferable for intended parents who are squeamish about the sight of blood or are concerned about being overwhelmed by the intensity of the birth. Delivery rooms aren't all that big, but putting yourself a few feet away from your surrogate mother might be the best place for you.

Of course you'll have to be mindful of any directions given to you by the doctor or nurses, and often they'll ask you to move or even help out with the delivery. Again, there's little about childbirth that's predictable! If you're clear on your surrogate's feelings on modesty as well as your wishes to participate in the birth, you're all much more likely to have a satisfying and memorable birth even when the unexpected arises.

Ask Yourself: Assuming the baby's delivery is progressing normally, from what vantage point would I most like to observe my baby's birth?

How does your surrogate mother feel about photos and videos during her labor and delivery?

Most women want some form of photo recording of their births, whether it's through pictures, or through videos, or a combination of both. Some women want every aspect (both the good and the bad) captured in pictures, while others prefer to have just the main highlights recorded. And while some surrogate mothers are comfortable with photos of their fully exposed bodies during the birth, others prefer more privacy.

Photos can be tricky because it's your baby who is being born, and you may want as many photos as possible of the birth. But birth pictures can also be highly personal, and your surrogate may feel more reserved and private about certain kinds of photos or videos.

Or it could be vice-versa—your surrogate may want more photos or videos of the birth (because even though it's your baby, it's her birth experience, too) and you may feel shy about taking very personal shots. If this is the case, you could have her husband take the more intimate photos and you can stick to ones that are not so graphic.

Along with discussing what photos or videos you do or do not want taken during the labor and delivery, it's important to talk about what each of you is comfortable sharing with family and friends after the birth. The same goes for sharing images on social media—discuss ahead of time what everyone is comfortable with.

Ask Yourself: Do my surrogate mother and I share similar views on photos and videos of the birth and if not, how can we compromise so we both feel respected and get what we want from the birth experience?

Is there something you envision about the birth that you'd like to see happen?

Chances are good that when you first thought about having a child, surrogacy was not the idea that initially popped into your mind. For most couples, using a surrogate is a wildly unexpected detour on the long road of infertility. So odds are good that you've constantly had to adjust and reevaluate your expectations along the way to parenthood.

But once your surrogate is pregnant and then as the pregnancy progresses and draws to a close, it's worth spending some time thinking about any particular desires that you have for the birth experience. Although your surrogate mother is the one who will physically give birth to your child, your baby's arrival into the world is your birth experience as well.

If all has gone well in your relationship with your surrogate mother throughout the pregnancy, you may have already discussed this in the previous nine months. Ideally, this is the case and there are no surprise expectations to negotiate as your baby's due date draws near. But things can change over time or feelings and yearnings can pop up, and it's important to acknowledge them and address them, if appropriate.

There's also nothing wrong with not having any particular hopes or expectations either—having an open mind and a flexible attitude is definitely a valuable asset when it comes to surrogacy. And truthfully, birth can be so unexpected and full of unanticipated events that sometimes having little to no preconceived notions is extremely helpful.

Ask Yourself: Do I have any hopes or expectations for the birth experience that my surrogate mother might be able to help fulfill and if so, have I clearly communicated them to her?

Where will you stay while your surrogate mother and baby are in the hospital?

During your surrogate's labor and delivery, it's most likely that you'll be spending the majority of your time all together in one room—probably the labor and delivery suite. Assuming that the birth is vaginal and uncomplicated, you'll also pass the next several hours immediately following the birth all together as your surrogate recovers and your baby is checked over by the doctor. These hours will probably fly by!

Once your surrogate moves to her post-partum recovery room, you too will need a space to settle in for the next day or so. Finding out what options are available to you from the hospital, as well as what your surrogate mother's preferences are, are all key factors in figuring out where you'll stay until you and your baby leave the hospital as a new family.

Some hospitals have enough empty rooms that you, your spouse, and your baby can have a room to yourselves until everyone is ready for discharge, which can be a nice option. This is always dependent on availability, and you have to be prepared for the event that there are no empty rooms available in the event of a baby boom. It makes good sense to have a hotel backup plan in place, even if you expect to stay at the hospital.

Some parents and surrogates elect to share one room for their stay, and enjoy passing the time together. Hospital room sizes can vary so it could be a very cozy couple of days, and it's possible that there's only space for one bed in the room, which your surrogate mother will be using. Usually there's a pull-out couch or a chair that reclines into a bed, but this will probably accommodate only one additional person. Be sure to find out the capacity of the postpartum rooms before your delivery date so you don't have any last minute surprises.

No matter if you plan to room in with your surrogate mother or have your own room nearby in the hospital, you'll need to meet with the hospital staff well in advance of the birth to explain your unique situation to them and find out what's available. They may or may not have had surrogate deliveries before, and each case can be different, and of course hospital policies, facilities and staff do change over time. They may assume you want the arrangements to be one way, only to find out you'd like something different, and they may be willing to accommodate you—you'll have to meet with them and ask.

Knowing what local hotel accommodations are available is smart regardless of where you plan to spend your time, because the unforeseen can always pop up. You may plan to spend all your time together with your surrogate mother and your baby until you're discharged, but your surrogate may have undergone an unplanned or emergency C-section and need peace and privacy to recuperate. Or your baby could experience complications and not be able to room in with you. It pays to come up with a plan that you'd prefer, but like anything else with pregnancy and birth, it also pays to keep a flexible attitude and have a back-up plan in mind as well.

Ask Yourself: Have I discussed plans and preferences for post-birth accommodations with both my surrogate mother and the hospital?

What are your plans for hospital visitors, both yours and your surrogate mother's?

For some families, birth is a huge celebration with family and friends streaming in just a few hours after the baby is born. Others prefer a quieter, more private first few days, soaking in their baby and the whole newness of parenting quietly by being alone until they leave the hospital. There is no right or wrong way, it's all about the experience that you and your surrogate mother would like to have during those first (and last!) few days together.

As always, hospital policy will dictate what visitors are allowed and when, so become familiar with the policy before your baby is born so you know the rules and the hours when visitors are accepted, if you'd like to have them.

If you have your own room at the hospital, your visitors will have little effect on your surrogate. But if you are sharing a room, or if you're staying in a hotel and passing the day in your surrogate mother's room in the hospital, you'll need to discuss any visitors with her. She may be open to any and all well-wishers coming by to meet the baby, or she may need more quiet downtime to recover.

Find out what her wishes are prior to labor, but also be mindful that the birth may not go as planned and you'll need to be flexible based on how your baby is doing and how your surrogate is recovering.

Unless she prefers otherwise, your surrogate's partner and children should be able to freely visit during her hospital stay, and they should be able to see, and if at all possible, hold the baby (depending on the ages of her children, of course). They have all seen her grow and care for this baby for the past nine months, and meeting the baby and seeing you with your new baby is a key part of them fully understanding the impact of the experience and reaching mental and emotional closure.

Your surrogate mother may want some private time with the baby as well, just to say goodbye in her own way. Even if you live close to each other and plan to visit frequently, it's an emotional transition for her to carry and birth your baby, then hand him or her off to you to take home. Even the most emotionally stable surrogate can get choked up at the intensity of the experience, so you have little reason to be concerned if she seems teary about the separation—she's got a lot of hormones in her body immediately after the birth! Unless you feel very uncomfortable with the idea, try to offer her some private time with the baby before you leave to go home.

Ask Yourself: Do I foresee visitors coming to the hospital, and how does my surrogate mother feel about having visitors besides her own immediate family?

How do you plan to leave the hospital when you're discharged?

Much of the way you leave the hospital will depend on the nature and time of the baby's birth, so you'll have to be flexible about your arrangements. However, it's worth thinking through and discussing what your ideal scenario might be, in case everything does happen to go according to plan (and in many cases, it does).

Most of the time the baby and surrogate mother are discharged from the hospital at the same time, but this is not universal. In some cases the surrogate's obstetrician will discharge her at a different time than the pediatrician discharges the baby, or the baby or surrogate may have some complications that require one of them to stay longer.

Assuming that everything has gone well and you're all discharged together, will you say your final goodbyes at the hospital? This will depend of course on if either of you need to travel any distance to get home. Will you be staying nearby before departing for home, and will you get together again before that time? Are there any particular photos that you or your surrogate mother wants to capture of the goodbye? Thinking through these questions ahead of time can help ease what is always a very emotional event.

Ask Yourself: How do I hope to say goodbye to my surrogate mother once the hospital stay is over?

Life After Baby's Birth

The birth of your baby is probably one of the greatest emotional highs you'll ever experience, and hopefully it's an equally positive one for both you and your surrogate mother. Once the birth is over, your journey as new parents, on your own and without your surrogate mother playing a role, begins. It's a very exciting time!

The vast majority of women who become gestational surrogates do it because they love the experience of pregnancy and childbirth, and they have a deep longing to help another woman become a mother or a couple become a family. They do not do it because they're longing for another baby themselves, in fact usually the opposite is true—they've moved onto a different phase of their lives where they no longer feel the yearning for a newborn.

However, your surrogate mother will definitely feel a connection to your baby. It's only natural, of course—she and your baby have been together for more than nine months and she's felt every hiccup, roll, and kick your baby made. Also, now that she's given birth, her postpartum hormones are in full effect and even she may be surprised by her feelings and emotions.

Knowing how you plan to handle communication and contact once your baby is born can be reassuring for both you and your surrogate mother, whether you hope for minimal contact or a great deal of contact. Of course it's impossible to entirely predict how the surrogacy experience will go for each of you, but talking over some of your post-birth hopes and expectations while still in the planning process is a good idea, to help avoid disappointment in the future.

Do you have any specific ideas about how much contact you'd like after the birth?

It can be hard to talk about specifics of post-birth contact when you are just getting to know each other or you're still in the early stages of the pregnancy, so it's not necessarily realistic to come to a firm agreement when you first meet. It is a topic worth broaching, though, to see if your views on contact are generally close to one another's. You would not want to agree to work with a surrogate mother who does not want any post-birth contact if you hope she attends the baby's birthday parties or other milestone events, and vice-versa. That would be setting up disappointment and discomfort for both of you.

Also, it's important to keep an open mind as life gets back to normal for all of you. You may find yourself wrapped up in caring for a newborn and with less free time than you imagined, and likewise, your surrogate mother may be enjoying returning to her usual day-to-day activities and family life. And it's hard to predict exactly how all of you will feel after the birth and how much time and energy you'll be able to devote to keeping up. Again, think through these issues to determine how you feel now and see how true those feelings seem as your baby's birth draws near.

Ask Yourself: How do I feel about keeping in touch immediately after the birth, and in the weeks and months to come? How do I feel about keeping in contact over the course of many years, or even a lifetime?

Are you open to sharing photos of your child with your surrogate mother? If so, how often?

Long gone are the days where new parents had to take photos with their camera, finish the roll of film, get the pictures developed and then mail the photos to their loved ones. Picture sharing has gone from a lengthy, expensive multi-step hassle to just the click of a button, quite literally.

Chances are that you'll be so smitten with your newborn baby that you'll be happy to text or email pictures frequently, and chances are also very good that your surrogate mother will appreciate these photos, even if you don't have time to send her a full update. She will look forward to watching your baby grow just the same as your own family does.

If you are not comfortable casually sharing photos with her, consider sending her yearly updates with pictures, perhaps near your baby's birthday. Regardless of whether or not you feel close to your surrogate or how close she feels to you, undoubtedly she feels close to the baby she gave birth to and would love regular updates and photos. If you know you don't want to share photos casually and frequently, you might let her know how often she might expect to receive a new picture of the baby.

Ask Yourself: Do I foresee an issue with sharing photos of my baby with my surrogate mother? If so, with what frequency am I comfortable with sharing them?

Are you open to visits in the coming months and years?

Again, the issue of post-birth contact is a complex one with lots of variables, including how close you live to each other, your family's schedule and obligations, your surrogate mother's family schedule and obligations, not to mention how the whole surrogacy experience went for all of you.

Some surrogacy arrangements, despite the best intentions on everyone's parts, do not end in a close relationship, and that's okay. There is no requirement that all of you remain close, lifelong friends (though a lot of intended parents and surrogates do go into the arrangement with this hope, and that's a lovely sentiment, too).

Like any other relationships in your lives, there will be ebbs and flows and the natural current of life will take over, even though the experience you've gone through together is one of the most profound ones you'll ever take part in. If you have any set feelings on future contact with each other, it's good to voice them as early as possible so everyone is clear and you can come to a middle ground of agreement, if necessary.

If you know going into surrogacy that you absolutely do not want any contact with your surrogate mother or contact between your surrogate and your child after the birth, it's important to express this upfront. There are surrogate mothers who can gladly accept these terms, while others are looking for more contact as the years go by, and either arrangement is fine, as long as everyone clearly knows upfront what it is. If you know definitively how you feel about future contact even before you begin the surrogacy process, discuss it with any potential surrogate mothers up front.

Ask Yourself: Knowing that things can change over the course of a gestational surrogacy experience, how do I feel today about maintaining contact with my surrogate as time goes by and my child grows? Is it something I welcome, or something I'd rather avoid?

Do you or your surrogate mother have any concerns about confidentiality regarding your identities and the surrogacy arrangement?

Most surrogacy contracts have a section about confidentiality and most of these requirements are boilerplate language rather than terms customized for each intended parent/gestational surrogate relationship. And for the most part this is fine, because as the pregnancy progresses and your relationship develops, you'll come to your own personal agreement that works for all of you. Much of the surrogacy process is governed by rules and procedures, but the influence of a growing personal relationship usually takes over contractual terms at some point.

The explosion of social media also makes the issue of confidentiality more complex, because information can very easily be shared, sometimes inadvertently. If you have concerns about how your information or pictures are shared with others, either through in-person conversation or on the Internet, talk to your surrogate mother about them. Some intended parents do not want to be identified by name, so surrogates will refer to them online using just their first initial, or perhaps a nickname or a pseudonym.

By the same token, ask your surrogate mother if she has any similar concerns about revealing her identity or sharing pictures of her. Most surrogate mothers are fine with information sharing, since they are proud of what they are doing and view the pregnancy and birth as a celebration to be shared, but don't assume this to be the case without asking her.

Also, if you have any concerns about your surrogate mother sharing photos of your baby, let her know. Most surrogates love to proudly share photos of the baby as it grows and most intended parents are proud to share as well, but if you feel differently, be sure to discuss it.

Some surrogacy agencies have very strict and specific guidelines for information and photo sharing so if this is the case for you, you'll have to defer to the terms of the agreement you have with the agency.

Ask Yourself: Are both my surrogate mother and I comfortable with sharing basic information about the surrogacy (in compliance with our legal agreement) or has our relationship evolved to something that allows for more liberal sharing, or perhaps less sharing?

What do you plan to tell the child about the circumstances of his or her birth? And at what age?

After struggling with infertility, it can seem a very long way into the future to have to worry about what to tell your child someday about the way he or she was brought into the world. And understandably, it can also be a difficult topic to think about when you're not even sure that your surrogate will get pregnant and you'll ever become parents.

Despite the unpredictability of the future, it's worth a little forethought on your part about what you'd like your child to know about his or her surrogate birth, and when. Some parents are open and forthright from the very beginning, even placing photos of the surrogate mother prominently in their home so the child knows from the beginning how he or she was born. Other parents are more reserved and choose to share the information about surrogacy once the child is old enough to ask about their own birth, and others don't want to reveal the circumstances of surrogacy at all.

Hopefully, during the course of your surrogate's pregnancy you will come to some clarity about how you want to handle the information with your child. When you do, be sure to share this information with your surrogate mother, so she can support your choice. Particularly, in this day and age of lightning-quick social media (and it's only going to get faster and more widespread), it's critical that everyone be on the same page regarding your wishes. While it may seem a silly thing to consider as you hold your newborn in your arms, time will fly and before you know it your child could come across information online that you didn't expect him or her to have access to.

Also, as your child gets a little older (say, age 4 or more) be sure to let your surrogate mother know what you've told your child about the birth. She should want to respect what you have or have not shared and if your child asks a question that catches her off-guard, she'll want to know what your child knows. Remember that surrogacy is the ultimate team sport, so the more information you can share, the better.

Ask Yourself: What do I want my child to know about the circumstances of his or her birth, and at what age? Do I want surrogacy to be part of the birth story from the first time my child hears it, or do I want to wait until my child is a bit older and better able to grasp the situation?

Summary

There is no question that taking part in gestational surrogacy can be one of the most intense and stressful experiences of your life, given all the unknowns in the process. And there is no guarantee at all that your surrogate will get pregnant and safely deliver your baby, though rapid medical advances make the chances of you holding your own newborn baby grow higher and higher each day.

Acknowledging the stress of the unknown that comes with infertility and gestational surrogacy, there are ways to ease the process for all of you by becoming fully informed of the surrogacy process. The process is unequivocally intense and complex, so understanding the nuances of the experience is the first step in growing a mutually beneficial, trusting and successful relationship. This guide gives you a lot to think through before searching for a surrogate mother, as well as questions and issues to explore together once you've met someone you're considering to take on the very special role as your surrogate mother.

There's little you can do to remove the anxiety and unpredictability of pregnancy and the process of birth. That's just the natural order of things. But you can prepare yourself for cultivating a relationship with your gestational surrogate that has the potential to be one of the most loving and rewarding experiences of your life, too.

I hope this guide has put you well on your way toward that.

Fertile and successful wishes to you!

The Successful Surrogacy Journal

Looking for some additional tips, inspiration, and a way to record your questions and thoughts before, during, and after your surrogacy experience?

I've put together a free companion journal just for you!

Print it out to record your thoughts in writing or type directly into the PDF—it's the perfect complement to this book.

Head to www.surrogacybydesign.com/journal to download The Successful Surrogacy Journal now!

About the Author

Susan MZ Fuller is a seven-time gestational surrogate mother who has delivered nine surrogate children over the course of twelve years. Her surrogacy experiences include two sets of twins, miscarriage, stillbirth, homebirth, waterbirth, two cesarean sections, and five subsequent vaginal births (VBACs). Her relationships with her intended parents have ranged from a distantly cool "business transaction" to intimately close and emotionally rewarding, and everything in between. She is the homeschooling mother of three and writes about her surrogacy experiences at surrogacybydesign.com.

Susan lives in Virginia, outside of Washington DC with her husband, children, and a menagerie of pets.

Visit her online at www.surrogacybydesign.com for articles and additional resources.

Made in the USA
Monee, IL
11 March 2021

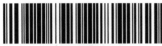

62487736R00049